The Fountain of Youth is Just A Breath Away: Breathing Exercises For Relaxation, Health And Vitality

Molly Larkin

Published by Four Winds Press

P.O. Box 176

Douglas, MI 49406

ISBN-13: 978-0692518069
ISBN-10: 0692518061

Contact: Molly Larkin   peace@mollylarkin.com

Front cover design: Jan Weren

"This is a fabulous book! It is clear, concise, and really helped me see how breathing can be an essential tool and important component in healing. Molly's enthusiasm is inspiring. After reading this book I was immediately able to begin a breathing practice and will share these gems with my clients."
~ Patricia Duncan, Counselor

"This marvelous little book on the benefits of breathing almost took my breath away! It is packed with gems of wisdom on the physical, mental, emotional, and spiritual aspects of breathing, along with well researched evidence to support the claim that breathing well is a direct path to fullness of well-being, and indeed, a fountain of youth. You owe it to yourself to buy and try this book!"
~ Rev. Rev. Marchiene Rienstra, Spiritual Leader, Interfaith Minister and Author of *Come to the Feast, Eisha's Search* and *The Future for Women*

"*The Fountain of Youth Is Just A Breath Away*, by Molly Larkin, is an insightful and practical approach to healthful breathing. Ms. Larkin encourages us to become conscious of our respiration and promises us rewards well beyond our efforts. This little book is packed with information that can transform your life."
~ Tobi Redlich, D.C., Yoga and Pranayama Instructor, Author of *Contemporary Runes: A Guide to Your Essential Self*

TABLE OF CONTENTS

Preface – Why This Book?

I never imagined I would write a book on breathwork, even though I've been an avid practitioner of breathing exercises for over 15 years.

I have read many books on breathing exercises, but I haven't found one that gave all the information I would love to see in one place. So I decided to write the book I've wanted to read.

My introduction to the importance of proper breathing was when I first took the course I now teach for the Healing in America School of Energy Medicine.

It's said that, *"When the student is ready, the teacher appears."*

A few weeks after taking the Healing in America course, I saw an article in the Los Angeles Times about the Art of Living Foundation, an organization that teaches classes in breathing exercises.

The timing was ideal – I took that class and have been doing daily breathing exercises every day since then.

Yes, every day for 15 years.

And I've reaped the benefits in improved health, emotional balance and peace of mind.

I have also been a student of yoga for well over 20 years, and any good yoga teacher will tell you that yoga is about the breath.

How has my daily practice changed me?

- I practice breathing exercises before my daily meditation– it helps prepare me for meditation because I start out calm, centered and feeling clearer.

- Alternate nostril breathing has balanced my brain and brought me peace of mind. I'm much calmer than I used to be in the face of challenges.

- I can take slower, deeper breaths than most anyone I know. [keep reading to find out why this is important]

- I enjoy absolutely excellent health at an age when most people's health is starting to decline.

- Last but not least, most people guess my age to be at least ten years younger than I actually am.

I would love that for you, too, so please read on to learn some breathing techniques that will improve your health, reduce your stress, promote peace of mind and help you live in the present moment.

Oh, yes, you may also feel as though you've discovered the Fountain of Youth!

INTRODUCTION

"If I had to limit my advice on healthier living to just one tip, it would be simply to learn how to breathe correctly." Andrew Weil, M.D.

What's the most urgent problem people are dealing with today?

Many would answer: stress.

In fact, the latest research says that at least 90% of all visits to the doctor are stress-related.

Yet, all too often, doctors prescribe the latest pharmaceutical for de-stressing[1], but there may be a better way.

Breathing exercises are one of the best solutions for invoking the *relaxation response* and thriving in life.

We all need to relax. Meditation is the most well-known relaxation technique, but many people have a hard time quieting their mind enough to feel they're actually meditating.

---

[1] This book, and the exercises described, are not meant to replace care by your physician. Check with a medical care provider or doctor before starting any breathing exercise practice.

Breathing exercises achieve the same level of relaxation, and at the same time, distract the mind because you have to focus on doing the exercise right. It's a clever way of tricking yourself into a meditative state without realizing it.

My first awareness of my breath

Some years ago I was a passenger in my boyfriend's car when he rear-ended the car in front of him, and we were immediately struck from behind.

The force of the impact propelled my body so hard into the shoulder belt it literally knocked the air out of me, leaving me gasping for breath.

In an attempt to take the focus off his having caused the accident, my boyfriend decided it would be a good idea to make fun of my gasping for breath and started making pretend gasping sounds himself.

Needless to say, I was neither comforted, nor amused.

Eventually my breath returned; and not long after, the boyfriend was gone.

Until one has an experience of being unable to breathe, it's easy to take the wonder of our breath for granted.

Perhaps it's the simplicity of breathing that leads us to forget its magnificence. We don't have to think about it; it just is.

But to the informed, just as we know that walking around the office or the house isn't enough exercise for our body [hence gyms, jogging shoes, bicycles and more], breathing exercises help counter our relatively sedentary lifestyles, supply our organs with oxygen necessary for health, and purge the body of toxins.

Mastering our breath can be the difference between thriving, or merely surviving, in life.

Chapter 1

SPIRITUAL ASPECTS OF THE BREATH

Many ancient cultures teach that life begins with the first inhale and ends with the last exhale. This is a profound truth, and yet we give very little thought to the breaths we take in between.

Why is that? Perhaps because we tend to take for granted all that is sacred around us.

Our breath is, indeed, sacred.

It can extend our lives, as well as the quality of our lives. It can calm us, focus our minds and bring life-giving oxygen into our body.

So, for a balanced, healthy life, it's time to start paying attention to it.

> *"The pause between breathing in and breathing out is the doorway to mystery."* Ojibway elder

All living organisms breathe.

Quite a few years ago, I sat on a hillside in Santa Monica, California and saw a mountain breathe. I literally saw, or imagined I saw, the mountain moving up and down, in and out. It gave me a profound experience of unity with all of creation.

That experience started me on my spiritual quest because it showed me that absolutely everything was alive and that we are all related to everything in creation.

Think about it. We are breathing the same air our ancestors breathed; the same air the spiritual masters such as the Christ and the Buddha breathed.

We are connected to every living thing through our breath. Everything breathes, and breathes with us.

We can survive weeks without food, days without water, and almost no time without breath. Yet most people use only a small part of their respiratory capacity. In fact, the typical person uses only 20% of their lung capacity!

Traditional Views Of The Breath

All ancient wisdom cultures understood the power of the breath, both as a physical necessity and a spiritual tool. It is central to the ancient practices of Yoga, Qi Gong, Tai Chi, Vipassana and many other meditative traditions.

Breath is Life – everything we inhale comes from the Universe.

In many cultures, the terms for "breath" and "spirit" are used interchangeably.

- In Sanskrit, the word *prana* means "breath, spirit or universal energy."

- In Latin, the word is *spiritus*.

- In Greek, the word for "spirit" is "*pneuma*" which also means "wind" or "breath."

- The ancient Hebrew word for God's Spirit is *Ruach*, which means breath.

- In Aramaic, the language spoken by the Christ, the word for Spirit includes breath, air and wind, and the term "Holy Spirit" can mean "holy breath."

According to Aramaic scholar Neil Douglas-Klotz in *The Hidden Gospel*, there is no separation in Aramaic between spirit and body or between humanity and nature. Our breath is connected to the air we breathe; therefore, in breath is unity with all beings.

In fact, Klotz says that the first line of The Lord's Prayer could be correctly translated from Aramaic as: "Respiration of all worlds, we hear you breathing – in and out – in silence."

Ancient Hindu masters called the human soul, "The one who breathes." They measured the span of a person's life, not in terms of how many years they lived, but in terms of the number of breaths they take from the moment they're born until the moment they die.

The chief spiritual discipline practiced by the Buddha was meditation on the breath. On his deathbed, in response to being asked what he'd gained by a lifetime of meditating on his breath, the Buddha said he had gained nothing, but, "I have lost my fear of sickness. I have lost my fear of old age, and I have lost my fear of death."[2]

In the indigenous purification lodge, water is poured on hot rocks to create heat and steam for the purpose of purifying body, mind and spirit. The steam created by the water poured on the rocks is called the "breath of Spirit."

Hildegard of Bingen, eight centuries ago, defined prayer as "breathing in and breathing out the one breath of the Universe."[3]

In yoga, Pranayama means breath control. [*Prana* means vital energy and *Yama* is self-control.]

Some teachers will say that the practice of yoga is really the practice of breath. Pranayama is actually a

---

[2] Caponigro p. 13-14

[3] Douglas-Klotz, *Prayers of the Cosmos*, intro

separate breathing practice to help clear the mind and cleanse the body.

Traditional Hawaiians use the term Haole [pronounced "Howlie"] to refer to non-Hawaiians – the term means "without breath," because when the Hawaiians first met Europeans they saw they were without Spirit or breath, meaning they had lost the ability to breathe naturally.

In fact, an ancient Hawaiian greeting is to touch foreheads together with hands clasped behind each other's head and actually exchange breath/Spirit together.

Chapter 2

A FEW BREATH FACTS

Each day we breathe about 20,000 times. In fact, the human body is designed to release 70% of its toxins through breathing. So it's important to get it right.

If we're not breathing fully:

- We're not ridding our bodies of all of its toxins through the breath and that means other systems in the body must therefore work overtime to do so. This in itself can lead to illness.[4]

- We're more easily fatigued due to reduced oxygen in the blood.

- We are less resistant to disease.

- Research suggests shallow breathing can cause sleep disorders, anxiety, stomach upsets, and more.

---

[4] Hendricks, p. 17

Benefits of Healthy Breathing

"Breathing is the basis for all our cellular functions, our energetic well-being, even our emotional health." Best-selling author and oncologist Mitchell Gaynor, M.D.

While your brain is only around three percent of your body mass, it can consume 20-30% of your body's oxygen intake. Its consumption increases during mental activities such as learning.

Each inhale brings in oxygen and starts the process of transforming our nutrients into fuel. Each exhale is a detoxification, releasing carbon dioxide. How we breathe can also affect our emotional state.

"Breath is like a natural masseuse," says Dennis Lewis in *The Tao of Natural Breathing*. "When we inhale fully, the diaphragm can … actually massage the stomach, liver, pancreas, intestines, and kidneys."

The movement of breath stimulates the lymphatic system, which is responsible for detoxifying the body. While the blood system has a pump [the heart], the lymphatic system has no pump other than our breath.

Research has shown that good breathing:

- Increases energy

- Lowers blood pressure

- Improves circulation

- Alleviates anxiety disorders without drugs

- Helps digestion

- Helps improve sleep

- Helps the nervous system to function more smoothly

- Can reduce pain

- Reduces stress

- Improves skin and reduces facial wrinkles

- Helps weight control as extra oxygen burns excess fat more easily

Pain Reduction Anyone?

During times of pain, the tendency is to have rapid, shallow breath, or even hold the breath, which actually can perpetuate pain.

Controlled, slow, gentle breathing can reduce the intensity of pain and help bring about relaxation.

Conscious abdominal breathing during childbirth helps to reduce the perception of pain.

Andrew Weil tells a story in his CD, *Breathing, the Master Key to Self-Healing*, of a trader on the Chicago stock market who got atrial fibrillation several times a year. It was usually treated with drugs until his doctor taught him a relaxing breath technique.

The next time his heart started beating irregularly, the trader did a relaxing breath; within 5 minutes his heart rate returned to normal and he was able to avoid going to the hospital.

The Breath, Illness and our Emotions

Our breath and emotions are so closely linked that we can actually change the way we feel by changing the way we breathe. Many people have been able to heal past emotions through breath without having to know anything about the original trauma. [5]

Eastern traditions, and knowledgeable holistic practitioners, understand that illness can sometimes start out as an emotional trauma stored in the body.

What happens when we experience emotional trauma? We often make a sharp intake of breath, then hold it. That intake and holding stores the trauma and anxiety in our bodies, where it may lie unnoticed for years until it eventually turns into illness.

---

[5] Caponigro p. 189

In the wild, animals will shake and snort after a trauma experience, shaking off the trauma with their movement and breath in order to return to homeostasis.

Andy Caponigro, in *Miracle of the Breath*, says that, "When we practice breath-balancing techniques, we're not only restoring the health of our breathing, we're also bringing our mood swings under control by changing the way we're breathing." [6]

Breathing techniques are a slow and gentle way of starting to release any blockages stored in the body.

Eastern philosophies have understood for thousands of years that slow, even breathing creates a sense of inner peace and well-being.

When we're stressed our breath becomes shallow and less oxygen gets to the brain, which may in turn signal the brain to go into panic mode.

It's helpful to do deep breathing before meditation or healing as it slows down the mind and helps us become more aware of our bodies.

If you don't have a meditation practice, focusing on slow, deep breathing is an excellent place to start.

---

[6] Caponigro p.190

You may even experience the magical feeling of *being breathed* by an unseen, Divine force!

Chapter 3

WHAT IS CORRECT BREATHING?

"Close to 80 percent of the Western population breathes incorrectly with habits such as breathing through your mouth instead of your nose, using the upper chest, and having noticeable breathing during rest." Dr. Joseph Mercola

The good news is that it's easy to learn to breathe correctly.

Healthy breathing practices are called natural, diaphragmatic, or abdominal breathing.

Abdominal breathing

Healthy abdominal breathing does not technically bring air into the abdomen. When the belly expands, the diaphragm contracts downward, which creates space for the lungs to fill. When the belly flattens on the exhale the diaphragm relaxes upwards, which deflates the lungs.

At the same time, the rib cage and lower back expand upon inhalation and contract the lungs on exhalation.

Steps to Conscious Breathing:

Step 1: Inhale slowly through the nose with a closed mouth, allowing your abdomen to rise, and the rib cage to expand.

Step 2: Exhale through the nose.

Practice this consciously throughout the day, making your breath deeper, slower, quieter and more regular.

If we become upset, our breath may become shallow, rapid, noisy and irregular. Changing how we breathe can change our physiology and may help to calm us down.

Ideally, in a person at rest, diaphragmatic breathing [through the nose only] should take place at a rate of 3-5 breaths per minute and the duration of the inhale is the same as the exhale.

Use a clock with a second hand to count how many breaths you take in a minute. One inhale and exhale makes one breath.

Most individuals at rest breathe at about 12-15 breaths per minute. That's much too fast, and much too shallow, for good health. [7]

---

[7] Fried, p. 28

Hyperventilation [abnormally fast breathing] is the most common of the stress-related disorders. It has been estimated to account for up to 60% of emergency ambulance calls in major U.S. cities. [8]

Until I began to study breathing techniques, I was a shallow breather, and I was known for frequent sighing, which can be a sign of abnormal breathing and stress. Scientists view too much sighing as a reset for breathing patterns that are getting out of whack; the sigh helps keep our respiratory system flexible.

I haven't sighed since I started daily breathing exercises.

PRACTICE: regularly practice abdominal breathing: [slow deep inhales so the belly rises, and exhales longer than the inhales as the belly contracts]. This will lead you to eventually breathe this way without trying.

The Healing Power of the Breath, or Why Exhales Should Be Longer Than Inhales

When your exhale is even a few counts longer than your inhale, the vagus nerve (which runs from the neck down through the diaphragm) sends a signal to your brain to turn up your parasympathetic nervous system [the relaxation response] and turn down your sympathetic nervous system [the stress response].

---

[8] Fried, p. 45

According to Lissa Rankin, M.D., the best selling author of *Mind over Medicine: Scientific Proof That You Can Heal Yourself,* the body's natural **self-repair mechanisms only work** when the relaxation response is activated.

Mouth v. Nose Breathing

We want to inhale through the nose for a number of reasons:

- There is a thin layer of protective mucous and tiny hairs [cilia] in the nasal passages which filter out at least 95% of dust particles, bacteria, and other airborne objects from reaching the lungs.

- Breathing through the smaller opening of the nostrils instead of the mouth gives us more control over our breath and tends to keep carbon dioxide in the body at the proper level. Because the nose is smaller than the mouth, nose breathing is a good vehicle to slow down the breath.

- Inhaling through the nose activates the parasympathetic nervous system [a good thing]. Breathing through the mouth increases the sympathetic nervous system [not a good thing].

- Because the nostrils are smaller then the mouth, air exhaled through the nose is slowed so the lungs have more time to extract oxygen from them. When there is proper oxygen-carbon dioxide exchange, the blood will maintain a balanced pH. If carbon dioxide is lost too quickly, as in mouth breathing, oxygen absorption is decreased. Therefore, slowing the breath through nose breathing contributes to more oxidation of the blood [up to 10-15%] and helps reduce stress.

- Breathing through the mouth allows airborne particles to go into the lungs, which can in turn stress the immune system and elimination organs.

- In yoga, nose breathing helps retain heat in the body, leading to warmed, loose muscles for added flexibility. This is why many yoga classes encourage nose breathing only.

Why do we tend toward shallow breath?

Surely one contributing factor to our overall shallow breath is our culture's obsession with beauty and flat abs!

Healthy, abdominal breathing involves letting our bellies expand to make room for the air and most people don't want their bellies to protrude.

Andrew Weil points out, "We're a country obsessed with flat stomachs. But tight, rigid abdominal muscles crimp the action of the diaphragm, which needs to move easily in order to breathe."

Natural abdominal breathing, which is what babies and animals do, involves fluid movement of the diaphragm, chest, ribs, belly and back. If you watch a baby sleeping, its belly naturally rises and falls with each breath. Simple.

However, the stress of life and the desire for six-pack abs has derailed us. Children today have lost the ability to breathe naturally by the age of six or seven. [9] That's when they start to take on stress and awareness of what adults are doing and they lose their natural ability for healthy breathing.

So we have to *re-learn* what we came into this life doing so well.

How do *YOU* breathe?

Place your left hand on your abdomen and your right on your chest. As you inhale, which hand moves more?

If your left hand moves more, you are an abdominal breather – congratulations!

If your right hand moves more, you are a chest breather and really need to study this chapter.

---

[9] Hendricks 58-59

Chest breathing is shallow and rapid, resulting in less oxygen to the blood and poor delivery of nutrients to the tissues.

Abdominal, or diaphragmatic, breathing is the healthiest way to breathe, and, with practice, you can train your body to breathe like this most of the time.

CAUTION: There may be conditions for which deep abdominal breathing may be contraindicated. Consult your doctor before beginning any breathing program if you are an insulin dependent diabetic, have metabolic acidosis or organ injury. [10]

Paying Attention to the Breath

There are traditions in Asia that say you can reach enlightenment by doing nothing other than paying attention to your breath.

Observation is a lost art in Western society, but it's how indigenous people for millennia knew where to find food, what weather was coming, and where danger lay.

Observation is the key to building intuition.

A good practice would be to observe your breath for 5 minutes once a day, sitting with a straight spine, eyes gently closed. If you don't yet have a meditation practice, this is a great place to start.

---

[10] Fried, p. 66

This can be done at any time; in the car, in the supermarket line, etc. In breathing therapy, patients learn to do slow, deep "abdominal breathing" at a rate of about 6 – 10 breaths a minute. That's a good goal!

Chapter 4

THE SCIENCE, or, as I like to call it, *Motivation*!

Numerous studies have directly associated respiratory capacity with longevity. The bottom line is that the better your lungs work, the longer you'll live.

The Busselton Health Study, a 13-year study conducted in Australia, demonstrated that respiratory capacity was a more significant factor than tobacco use, cholesterol levels, and insulin metabolism in determining people's longevity.

The 29-year-long Buffalo Health Study found a direct correlation between lung function and longevity. The follow-up study published in the journal *Chest* in 2000, concluded that "pulmonary function is a long-term predictor for overall survival rates in both genders and could be used as a tool in general health assessment."

The Framingham Heart Study, also a 30-year study which started in 1948, is one of the largest and most renowned medical studies ever performed, and forever changed the way the medical community views the progression of disease. Following 5,200 people from Framingham, Massachusetts for over three decades, one of its startling conclusions was the determination that the **greatest predictor of health and longevity is lung volume**.

Over our lifetime, our respiratory capacity naturally decreases unless we are consciously working to maintain it. The Framingham Study determined that the average person reaches peak respiratory function and lung capacity in their mid-20s, after which they start to lose up to 9 – 27% of their lung capacity each decade of their life.

In fact, the **average person uses only 20% of their lung capacity**!

It's believed that diminished respiratory capacity is one of the reasons the elderly so easily succumb to pneumonia.

Dr. Otto Warburg received the 1931 Nobel Prize for proving that cancer cells are anaerobic, meaning they cannot survive in an oxygen-rich environment. Germs, fungi and bacteria are also anaerobic.

Lack of oxygen reserves is also a risk factor in heart attacks.

In a nutshell, the better you breathe, the longer and better you live.

Now that's worth doing something about!

Chapter 5

ANATOMY LESSON

While helpful in understanding the importance of breathing, this next section is rather technical. If this is too technical for you, skip ahead to Chapter 6.

Diaphragm: this is a large muscle located between the chest and the abdomen.

Intercostal muscles: these are several groups of muscles that run between the ribs and help form and move the chest wall. They help expand and shrink the size of the chest cavity when you breathe.

Breathing influences the **autonomic nervous system [ANS],** which regulates blood pressure, heart rate, circulation, digestion, and more. It's also called the involuntary nervous system because it controls those things we don't have to consciously think about in order for them to function. Many modern illnesses, such as high blood pressure, are related to nervous system imbalances.

The autonomic nervous system has two components:

First, **the sympathetic nervous system** controls heart rate, blood pressure, breathing rate, and pupil size, and causes blood vessels to narrow and decreases digestive juices. This is the **"Fight or flight"** part of the nervous system that takes over when you meet a lion on the savannah and have to run for your life.

Next**, the parasympathetic nervous system** comes into play during **rest and relaxation:** it slows the heart, dilates blood vessels, decreases pupil size, increases digestive juices, and relaxes muscles in the gastrointestinal tract.[11] [12]

The human body was not built for today's sedentary lifestyle. It used to be nothing to walk twelve miles and that would work off our stress. We have no comparable way to work it off today; we're simply not as active as we were built to be.

Many people today have illnesses attributable to nervous system imbalances. We are confronting modern problems with a nervous system designed to live on the savannah.

On the savannah, when the lion gives up on chasing us and walks away, our nervous system returns to rest after we also walk around to release the trauma of the chase. It also gives the body time to get the breath back to normal.

---

[11]http://www.americanheart.org/presenter.jhtml?identifier=4463

[12] http://www.cancer.gov/dictionary

In a modern life of continuous stress, there's no such balance to be had.

We're in a constant state of alarm because of all the conflict and fear we take in by watching the news, television and movies. The trauma and horror is going into our bodies and we're stuck with it.

High blood pressure is one result of modern day stressors and our response to it.

Most of us can't consciously slow our heart rate, lower blood pressure, relax our muscles and decrease perspiration, BUT, the breath can be used to control these things by influencing the parasympathetic nervous system into a relaxation response.

In addition, I believe one reason people smoke is that it changes their breathing and relaxes them. We can relax by changing our breathing without the use of tobacco.

Chapter 6

CHANTING, TONING AND THE BREATH

There's a great deal of interest in toning and sound healing today.

Interestingly, of all the sound-making devices and instruments found on this planet, the instrument we are born with, the human voice, is believed by many to have the most healing qualities.

Toning and chanting, the use of the voice to create sound, is the oldest and most natural form of sound healing.

Toning uses non-verbal sounds [i.e., no words]. Chanting includes words.

Our voice was the first healing instrument. When you hurt yourself and moan or say, "ow, ow, ow," you're actually doing sound healing!

In the late 1960s, a French physician, Alfred Tomatis, was called in to a Benedictine monastery in the south of France because many of the monks were suffering from rare and undiagnosed symptoms: they were inexplicably exhausted.

Other physicians were stumped so they called in Dr. Tomatis. He discovered that in the wake of Vatican II reforms instituted by the Catholic Church in the mid-1960s, the new abbot decreed the brothers should abandon their traditional practice of singing Gregorian chants 6-8 hours a day.

Tomatis, who has been called the "Einstein of sound," surmised that the chanting had functioned as a way to energize the monks by "awakening the field of their consciousness." He suggested they start chanting again; they did so and within five months they were fully recovered. [13]

Research on toning and chanting

Dr. Mitchell Gaynor's clinical experience is that chanting can synchronize the brain waves to achieve profound states of relaxation.

Research by Dr. David Simon, Medical Director of the Chopra Center for Well-Being reveals that healing chants and music have measurable physiological effects.

Simon has found that chants are "chemically metabolized into endogenous opiates" that are both internal painkillers as well as healing agents in the body. [14]

---

[13] Gaynor, p. 13
[14] Gaynor, p. 18

Music also has a powerful positive influence on the protective cells of the immune system, which fight invading pathogens and perform the task of regenerating injured tissues. [15]

The languages of many ancient cultures are considered spiritual languages, which includes the belief that they create a vibration in the body that helps bring about healing.

Examples would be Sanskrit, Lakota, Hebrew and Arabic. And based on my experience, the Hopi language would be yet another.

I recall attending a ceremony at a Hopi village many years ago. Men dressed as kachinas entered the square chanting in a deep voice that almost sounded as though it came from under the ground.

The sound in turn created a vibration in those standing and watching, and I have no doubt that it was a healing vibration.

Much indigenous healing involves chanting. Some tribes perform healing with herbs over which they first chant. I've come to understand that the chant serves three functions:

1. It serves as an instruction to the herb to tell it how to function in the body.

2. The chant also changes the vibrational

---

[15] Gaynor, p. 18

frequency of the herb so that it becomes exactly what is needed to repair a particular illness.

3. The herb then changes the vibrational frequency of the ill/injured part of the body to bring it back to health.

I mention chanting and toning because some of the breathing techniques in this book will involve chanting. So you'll have a combination of the best of both worlds: breath and sound!

Chapter 7

WHAT YOUR DOCTOR MAY NOT KNOW CAN HURT YOU

or,

don't wait for your doctor to teach you how to breathe

Psychologist and breathing instructor Gay Hendricks, Ph.D. tells this intriguing but frustrating story involving a study of a rare lung disease that took place at Stanford University in the 1980s. At the time, there was no known cure for the disease.

One of the women in the study had the insight that learning correct breathing techniques might help her, so she asked the research team to teach her to breathe better. No one knew what to tell her!

They also thought it was odd for her to want to learn how to breathe.

She researched breathing on her own and found a doctor who taught her some breathing exercises. Within a month, the lung disease had disappeared.

And it never returned.

The research team recorded her cure as "spontaneous remission" and expressed no interest in learning what she had done to bring it about.[16]

Hendricks reports that many physicians tell him they get extensive training in respiratory disease, but little training on how to identify or teach effective breathing.

Mitchell L. Gaynor, M.D., uses music, vocalization, breathing and meditation techniques in his work with critically ill patients. He points out that most medical students learn little or nothing about the complexities and subtleties of the breath.[17]

The Birmingham Assessment of Breathing Study [BABS], published in 2005, was conducted at the University of Birmingham in England. The study aimed to test the ability of medical students to discriminate between normal and abnormal breathing patterns in order to select the correct course of treatment.

The study concluded that medical students were unable to reliably distinguish between normal and abnormal breathing, resulting in a high number of inappropriate, potentially harmful actions.

Gaynor says that, "If I were organizing a medical curriculum, I would start by teaching future doctors to learn how to breathe."

---

[16] Hendricks, p. 15
[17] Gaynor, p. 56

I've referred previously to Dr. Andrew Weil, Director of the Center for Integrative Medicine of the College of Medicine, University of Arizona where, you guessed it, breath work is part of the curriculum. Let's hope that will be only the beginning of a national trend in medical schools.

Chapter 8

THE BREATHING EXERCISES

Ease into these practices. Don't do them all in one sitting. Practice one or two a day, for no more than a few minutes, otherwise you could feel lightheaded.

Our brains are not used to being well oxygenated so we need to work our way up to 15 minutes of breathwork each day.

Make a regular practice of the ones you enjoy. When you read the section on the chakras, you may choose the techniques that will work on opening and healing specific areas.

All breathing exercises should be done while sitting with a straight spine.

A Basic Exercise for Abdominal Breathing[18]

This is the most important and basic breath to master first. If you practice nothing else in this book, please learn this one.

18

http://www.amsa.org/healingthehealer/breathing.cfm

1. Place one hand on the abdomen, and the other on your chest. Take a deep, slow inhale through the nostrils, making sure the abdomen expands out more than the chest. This ensures that the base of the lungs are getting air.

2. Exhale.

3. Inhale through the nose to a count of 7, letting the abdomen rise.

4. Slowly exhale to a count of 8, while contracting your abdominal muscles to assist the expulsion of air.

5. Repeat this cycle four more times for a total of 5 deep inhales/exhales. You ideally want to work up to breathing at a rate of one breath every 10 seconds [or six breaths a minute].

It takes time and practice for this to feel comfortable, and will be more than worthwhile to achieve. Ultimately, work toward the exhales being twice as long as the inhales.

We deepen inhalation through extending our exhalation. This makes room for more air to come in to our lungs.

Simple Meditative Breath

1. Close your eyes; and make sure your spine is straight.

2. Pay attention to your breath for 10 breaths as you inhale and exhale.

3. Try to make the exhale longer – the more you exhale, the more room there is for the next inhale. A well-functioning body relies on taking in oxygen and releasing carbon dioxide.

Work your way up to 5 minutes a day, increasing the number of breaths each day.

Now we move into the slightly more complex techniques:

Alternate Nostril Breathing: [Nadi shodhana]

Benefits: Alternate nostril breathing enhances brain balance. It stimulates the brain, brings alertness, and calms the nervous system. It also activates the 6th chakra, which is the gateway to intuition.

A little known fact about our nostrils is that we naturally breathe through predominantly one nostril at a time and every couple of hours it switches over to the other side. This process helps to balance the right and left hemispheres of the brain. A balanced brain optimizes creativity, logic, and verbal ability.

Yogis consider this one of the best techniques to balance the mind and nervous system. I have practiced alternate nostril breathing for over 15 years on a daily basis and truly believe it has helped me to become calmer and more balanced.

<u>How to do it</u>:

The breath should be slow and inaudible in this exercise.

> 1. Use your right thumb to close off your right nostril.
>
> 2. Inhale slowly through left nostril.
>
> 3. Pause for a second.
>
> 4. Now close left nostril with your left ring finger and release your thumb from the right nostril.
>
> 5. Exhale through your right nostril.
>
> 6. Now, inhale through right nostril.
>
> 7. Pause.
>
> 8. Use right thumb to close the right nostril.
>
> 9. Breathe out through left nostril.

These nine steps make up one cycle. In the beginning, this technique should be done no more than three complete cycles at one time. Daily practice is ideal; add one round a week and make your breath as slow as possible.

Try to work up to five rounds per minute. Since most people breathe 12-15 times per minute, this will be a nice, slow pace which will maximize building lung capacity. Remember that healthy breathing is 5-6 breaths per minute; 12-15 breaths per minute is way too shallow.

When first starting breathing exercises, do not do them longer than advised. Deep breathing exercises oxygenate the brain and can cause lightheadedness when we're not used to it. Work up to it, as with any exercise.

Sit quietly for a few moments after you have finished.

Caution: Do not practice this breath if you have a cold or your nasal passages are blocked. Do not hold your breath if you have high blood pressure. More advanced methods of alternate nostril breathing need to be practiced with an experienced practitioner. Practicing on an empty stomach is preferred.

4-4-6-2 breath

Benefits: lowers anxiety.

Over the years I have come across other inhale/hold/exhale breaths, with a variety of timing patterns. They all work, when done as instructed.

What's important is to retain breath between the inhale and the exhale, giving your body time to use the oxygen.

How to do it:

1. Begin by exhaling fully.

2. Inhale through both nostrils to a count of **four.**

3. Hold the breath for a count of **four.**

4. Exhale to a count of **six**.

5. Hold for **two**.

Repeat.

The ratio is what's important, not the length of your count.

Complete only four rounds of this exercise at one sitting and do it no more than twice a day before increasing. Again, your brain isn't used to being oxygenated; it's good for it, but you have to build up to it to avoid getting light headed. I recommend working up to five minutes of this breath.

4-7-8 Breath

Benefits: This is currently being touted as a wonderful sleep aid.

Sit with your back straight when first practicing it, but ultimately it can be done lying down, too.

How to do it:

1. Start with an exhale.

2. Inhale quietly [through the nose, with mouth closed] to a count of four.

3. Hold for a count of seven.

4. Exhale [audibly thru mouth, tongue at back of teeth, making a whoosh sound] for a count of eight.

The ratio is what's important, not the length of your count.

Do this breath only four times at one sitting, and no more than twice a day before increasing. Your brain isn't used to being oxygenated; it's good for it, but you have to build up to it to avoid getting light headed.

We've already learned that inhaling then holding the breath leads to an overall increased level of oxygen in the body. The more oxygen in your system, the less work for your body to do.

Also, remember that longer exhales help your body relax and unwind.

Stimulating Breath [also known as **Breath of Fire**]

Benefits: If you need a pick-me-up or are feeling a bit anxious, try the Stimulating Breath; it can help energize and clear your mind.

When you first begin, try it for just 15 seconds, increasing the duration by five seconds every time until you can complete one full minute. Always breathe normally between exercises.

How to do it:

1. Sit upright with your back straight, eyes closed, and shoulders relaxed.

2. Place the tip of your tongue against the bony ridge behind and above your upper teeth.

3. Breathe rapidly through your nose, in and out, with your mouth slightly closed.

4. Keep your inhale and exhale short and equal. Your chest should be almost mechanical in its movements - moving air rapidly, like a manual bicycle pump.

5. Try to inhale and exhale three times per second, if you can, keeping your breath audible.

Ideally, you will feel the muscular effects of this breathing exercise at the base of your neck (just above the collarbone) and at the diaphragm. Put your hands on these areas to get a sense of the movements.

Humming Bee Breath [aka **Brahmari**]

Benefits:
- stimulates the pituitary gland and third eye,
- reduces stress,
- increases relaxation.

The pituitary is the master gland for the endocrine system. Stimulating and balancing the pituitary through the Bumble Bee Breath will in turn help regulate the endocrine system, balancing hormones and blood sugar.

How to do it:

1. Start, as always, in a comfortable seated position with a straight spine.

2. Block your ears by placing your thumbs lightly over them.

3. Place your index fingers above your eyebrows.

4. Place your two middle fingers over your closed eyelids.

5. Place your pinky fingers against the sides of your nostrils [do not close the nostrils with your

fingers, just let them lightly rest there].

6. With your mouth closed, inhale through the nose.

7. With a closed mouth, exhale through the nose while making a low humming sound in your throat, like a bee.

8. Hum during your exhale until there is no breath left, then repeat.

You will feel the sound vibration throughout your head. Practice this for 2-3 minutes.

Precautions:
Only perform while seated, never lying down.
Do not perform if you have an ear infection.
Do not perform after eating a heavy meal.
As with all breathing exercises, if you feel lightheaded, stop!

Brahma Mudra [Ah-oo-ee-mm breath]

Benefits: This breathing technique opens the throat chakra.

How to do it:

1. Inhale through the nose while turning your head to look over the right shoulder; turn your head back to center while exhaling and chanting a slow long "ah."

2. Inhale through the nose while turning your head to look over the left shoulder; turn your head back to center while exhaling and chanting a slow long "oo."

3. Inhale through the nose while turning your head up as if to look at the sky; bring your head back to center while exhaling and chanting a slow long "eee."

4. Inhale while lowering your head to look down; bring your head back up to level while slowly exhaling and humming "mmmmm."

Repeat this series no more than 2-3 times at the beginning.

Heart Opening Breath

Breathing originates in the chest, which is the area of the heart and lungs. Blockages here can result in asthma, shortness of breath, lung disease, heart disease and high blood pressure.

The heart is also the connection and integration point between the upper and lower chakras, so opening this area will allow for greater connection between body and mind.

How to do it:

1. Sit with your spine straight, breathing slowly and deeply.

2. Keep your eyes closed.

3. Extend your arms straight out in front of you, palms and fingers together as in prayer, pointing in front of you, parallel to the floor.

4. Open your arms wide as you inhale, bringing your shoulder blades as close together as possible. Visualize your heart center opening and expanding as you fill your lungs with air.

5. With the expansion, silently say, "I open my heart to give and receive love."

6. With your straight arms still parallel to the ground, exhale and bring your arms and hands back to the original position, in front of you,

palms together.

7. Keep a slow and steady pace, being gentle with your heart.

8. Repeat 26 times[19], with your eyes closed.

Washing Machine Breath

Benefits: This enhances the solar plexus chakra and cleanses the liver.

1. Sit cross-legged on the floor or on a stool with your spine straight, feet flat on the floor. [Don't use a chair with a back because it will likely get in the way of your movement.]

2. Raise both arms in the goal post position and have the pointer finger and thumb of each hand touching.

3. On an inhale through the nose, rotate your entire body at the waist to the left; on an exhale, rotate to the right.

4. Go back and forth like this for 30-60 seconds.

---

[19] Twenty-six repetitions is common in Kundalini Yoga, because we have twenty-six vertebrae in the spine. Gurmuck, p. xxxi.

This exercise literally cleanses the liver – it's like squeezing water out of a wet sponge. [The liver is your body's primary detoxification organ.]

The New CPR

I would be remiss if I didn't include this fascinating modification to the traditional method of CPR [cardiopulmonary resuscitation].

In a major change, the American Heart Association said in 2008 that hands-only CPR — rapid, deep presses on the victim's chest until help arrives — works just as well as standard CPR for sudden cardiac arrest in adults.

This means you can skip the mouth-to-mouth breathing and just press on the chest to save a life – ironically, it's most effective to do it in time to the classic BeeGee's song, *Stayin' Alive*.

The reason this works is that when an adult collapses from cardiac arrest, they still have ample air in the lungs and blood. Compressions will keep the blood flowing to the brain, heart and other organs.

Caution: Do this for heart attacks only, not drowning or trauma.

Chanting OM

OM is known as the universal sound of perfection. Chanting OM vibrates at the frequency of 432 hz, which is the vibrational frequency of everything in nature. So it is the sound of the universe.

There is a reason many yoga classes begin and end with the chanting of OM. OM is the most universally used chant for opening and balancing the chakras; it connects us to the infinite vibration from which our universe is comprised.

Buddhist scriptures reveal that OM is the most powerful sound, that its power alone can bring enlightenment.

Scientists have recorded the sound of the earth spinning on its axis and it's the sound of OM.

How to chant OM

1. Chanted correctly, it consists of three syllables: A, U, M.

2. The first syllable, A, is pronounced as a long "aw." As you start at the back of your throat, expect to feel a vibration in your chest.

3. The second syllable, U, is pronounced as a long "oo." Your throat should vibrate as you make this sound.

4. The third syllable, M, is pronounced as a long

"mmmmm" with your tongue gently touching the back of your front teeth.

5. Inhale through the nose, and exhale while chanting OM. When your breath ends, pause ever so briefly and repeat.

6. Seven OMs in a row is a good place to start. When done together with a group of people, as in a yoga class, it creates a very powerful vibration. It also sets you up for an excellent meditation.

Chapter 9

HEALING THE CHAKRAS THROUGH THE BREATH

What are the chakras; why should you care?

Everything in our world is made up of energy; including our physical bodies. Our bodies have energy centers, known as "chakras," which are how we exchange energy with the world around us.

The term "chakra" comes from the Sanskrit language and means "spinning wheel," because clairvoyants can see them spinning. That makes sense, since energy always moves.

Healthy chakras spin in a clockwise direction. If the chakra spins counterclockwise or in a shape that is not in a circle, it could be an indication of an imbalance in the energy field.

It's important to keep our energy fields clear and balanced so that physical illness doesn't manifest.

It is generally acknowledged that humans have 7 main chakras [some systems claim more than 7 main chakras] and hundreds of minor chakras, but we'll stick with 7 for the purposes of this book.

They are all access points for energy to flow into and out of the energy fields of the human body.

"It is important to open the chakras and increase our energy flow, because the more energy we let flow, the healthier we are. Illness in the system is caused by an imbalance of energy or a blocking of the flow of energy." [20]

Sometimes, in the quest to increase their spirituality, people want to focus only on the heart, third eye or crown chakras. However, to lead a balanced life, which is at the core of spirituality, all of the chakras need to be balanced. Breathing exercises can help to do that.

Here is a brief overview of the 7 main chakras, with an explanation of what they help us with:

[Note: Different modalities of energy healing may associate different colors or organs with the chakras; the following chart is what most systems seem to agree to.]

---

[20] Brennan, p. 45.

Chakra	Color	Associated psychological function	Associated organ	Recommended Breathing technique
Crown	Violet	Spirituality, Connection with a Higher Power	Pineal gland	Chant OM
Third Eye	Indigo	Intuition; mental functioning	Pituitary gland	Humming Bee Breath
Throat	Blue	Communication	Thyroid	Brahma Mudra Chant OM
Heart	Green	Love and compassion	Thymus	Heart Opening Breath Chant OM
Solar Plexus	Yellow	Self-esteem; emotional balance; knowing our place in the universe	Pancreas	Washing Machine Breath
Sacral	Orange	Sexual energy, creativity, joy	Adrenals	Diaphragmatic breathing, Focusing on breathing through the tailbone and hips.
Root	Red	Sexuality; connection to our ancestors, safety, grounding	Gonads	Diaphragmatic breathing, focusing on breathing through the tailbone and hips.

Breathing Exercises To Open And Balance The Chakras

Good breathing feeds light into the chakras and helps keep them open and balanced. I think you can see from the above explanation that keeping the chakras open and balanced is a really good practice. So this section includes breathing exercises specific to each chakra.

If you have an emotional or physical issue going on that is associated with one particular chakra, breathing exercises for that chakra may help facilitate healing.

For example, if you are feeling sadness due to a relationship issue, healing the heart chakra may be in order. Therefore, practice the heart opening breath.

If you are have having trouble expressing yourself to a colleague, practice an exercise for the throat chakra.

And so on.

Just a reminder: All breathing exercises should be done while sitting with a **straight spine**.

[Note: When sitting on the floor, it can be a good practice to sit on a yoga block or pillow so that the hips are higher than the feet. This is a more comfortable position, and assists in keeping the spine straight].

The Breathing Techniques for Each Chakra

Crown Chakra: Chant OM

Third Eye – Humming Bee Breath

Throat: There are two breathing techniques that can open and balance the throat chakra and stimulate the thyroid. Do either one or both:

- Brahma Mudra [Ah-oo-ee-mm breath]

- Alternatively, chant OM.

Heart:

- Chant OM – stimulates heart and thymus

- Heart opening breath

Solar Plexus: Washing Machine Breath

Root And Sacral: Diaphragmatic breathing, focusing on breathing through the tailbone and hips.

The root chakra connects us to the earth, our ancestors and our tribes. It deals with issues of safety and protection. If we learn to trust that the inhale will always follow the exhale, we will have enhanced our trust.

CONCLUSION

Not only is breathing important to our health, it is vital to reaching higher levels of consciousness. It is also an excellent step on the path to starting a regular meditation practice, which can expand our inner awareness and spiritual connection.

"Air is a living being. Air welcomed you into your life with your very first breath. Air is the very last living being that you will say good-bye to as you leave this life with your last breath." [Sandra Ingerman in *Walking in Light: the Everyday Empowerment of a Shamanic Life, p. 57.*]

Let's get to know air well during the life in between.

Breathing is the first and last thing we do in life. Cherish it!

REFERENCES

Brennan, Barbara, *Hands of Light; A Guide to Healing Through the Human Energy Field.* Bantam Books, 1987.

Caponigro, Andy, *Miracle of the Breath; Mastering Fear, Healing Illness, and Experiencing the Divine.* New World Library, 2005.

Douglas-Klotz, Neil, *The Hidden Gospel*, Quest Books, 2012.

Douglas-Klotz, Neil, *Prayers of the Cosmos; Meditations on the Aramaic Words of Jesus.* Harper Collins, 1990.

Fried, Robert, Ph.D *Breathe Well, Be Well; A Program to Relieve Stress, Anxiety, Asthma, Hypertension, Migraine, and Other Disorders.* New World Library, 1999.

Gaynor, Mitchell, M.D., *The Healing Power of Sound; Recovery from Life-Threatening Illness Using Sound, Voice and Music.* Boston: Shambhala 2002.

Gurmukh with Cathryn Michon, *The 8 Human Talents; Restore the Balance and Serenity Within You with Kundalini Yoga.* Harper Collins, 2000.

Harrold, Ed, "Find health with your breath – The Nose is for breathing and the mouth is for eating." *Natural News*, August 16, 2011, http://www.naturalnews.com/033332_health_breath.html

Hendricks, Gay, Ph.D., *Conscious Breathing; Breathwork for Health, Stress Release, and Personal Mastery*, Bantam Books, 1995.

Ingerman, Sandra, *Walking in Light; the Everyday Empowerment of a Shamanic Life*. Sounds True, 2014.

Knuiman, MW; James, AL; Divitini, ML; Ryan, G; Bartholomew, HC; Musk, AW, "Lung Function, respiratory symptoms and mortality: results from the Busselton Health Study." http://www.ncbi.nlm.nih.gov/pubmed/10976856.

Lewis, Dennis, *The Tao of Natural Breathing; for Health, Wellbeing and Inner Growth.* Berkley: Rodmell Press, 2006.

Miller, Julie Ann, "Overview of the Groundbreaking FRAMINGHAM STUDY on LONGEVITY and BREATHING --Making Old Age Measure Up." *Science News*. Vol. 120, August 1, 1981. http://www.breathing.com/pdf/makingoldagemeasureup.pdf.

Perkins GD, Stephenson B, Hulme J, Monsieurs KG. "Birmingham assessment of breathing study

(BABS)." *Resuscitation.* 2005; 64(1):109-13.
[PUBMED ID 15629563].

Rankin, Lissa, M.D., *Mind Over Medicine: Scientific Proof That You Can Heal Yourself.* Hay House, 2014.

Schunemann, Holger J. M.D., Ph.D.; Dorn, Joan, Ph.D.; Grant, Brydon J. B. M.D., F.C.C.P.; Winkelstein, Warren Jr., M.D., M.P.H.; and Trevisan, Maurizio, M.D., M.S., "Pulmonary Function is a Long-term Predictor of Mortality in the General Population: 29-Year Follow-up of the Buffalo Health Study."
CHEST. 118(3) © 2000 American College of Chest Physicians, 09/01/2000.

Weil, Andrew, *Breathing, the Master Key to Self-Healing*, Audio Book, Sounds True, 2001.

About the Author

Molly Larkin has been a spiritual seeker and student of human potential since the age of seven, when her teacher said human beings only use 10% of their brain capacity. She decided then and there to learn to use 100% of hers, a decision which led her on a life-long spiritual quest.

She is the co-author, with Muskogee Creek elder Marcellus "Bear Heart" Williams, of the international best-seller *The Wind Is My Mother; the Life and Teachings of a Native American Shaman.*

She has studied with indigenous elders from around the world for over 30 years. Her passion for health and healing led her to become a certified healing practitioner and Licensed Trainer for <u>Healing in America</u>.

In her private healing practice, Molly works with people, pets and horses, helping them achieve emotional, spiritual and physical balance.

You can receive ongoing teachings and inspiration by subscribing to her blog, "Ancient Wisdom for Balanced Living," at www.MollyLarkin.com.